Polio Lame

A Handbook On The History, Prevention and Treatment of Polio

Dr. Susan Berger

Dedication

Dedicated to all those that have been rendered lame due of this deadly disease

Table of content

Chapter 1: What is polio

A virus is the cause of the potentially fatal condition polio. Poliovirus is the illness known as polio (or poliomyelitis). It can be fatal and result in permanent paralysis (inability to move certain body parts).

The frequency of polio cases worldwide has decreased by 99% since 1988. Since 1979, there hasn't been a polio outbreak in the US. 33 instances were recorded globally in 2018, according to sources. While many nations have eradicated polio, some still do. And anyone who is not immune to the virus and comes into touch with it can get it. To make sure individuals are inoculated is the most effective strategy to eradicate polio for good worldwide.

Polio History

As it paralyzed hundreds of thousands of children each year, polio was one of the most dreaded illnesses in industrialized nations at the turn of the 20th century. However, polio was quickly brought under control and essentially eradicated as a public health issue in these nations in the 1950s and 1960s with the development of efficient vaccinations.

From 1580 B.C. until the present, you may follow the progression of polio by using this interactive timeline.

It took some time for polio to be acknowledged as a serious issue in poor nations. Surveys on lameness conducted in the 1970s showed that the condition was also common in emerging nations. As a result, regular vaccination became a feature of national immunization programs in the

1970s, which helped many developing nations manage the illness.

In 1985, Rotary International began a global campaign to immunize children throughout the world against polio. In 1988, the Global Polio Eradication Initiative (GPEI) was established. At the time of the GPEI, polio paralyzed more than 1000 children daily around the world. With the help of more than 200 nations and 20 million volunteers, more than 2.5 billion children have received the polio vaccine since that time.

Only two nations still have wild poliovirus in circulation today, and the incidence of polio cases worldwide has dropped by 99%.

Additionally, some strains of the virus have been successfully eradicated; of the three types of wild polioviruses (WPVs), type 2's last case was reported in 1999, and its eradication was announced in September 2015; type 3's most recent case dates to

November 2012, and this strain was declared to be completely eradicated in the world in October 2019.

A debilitating and perhaps deadly viral illness, polio. Although there is no cure, there are secure and reliable immunizations. In order to prevent infection, every kid must receive the polio vaccine until transmission ceases and the globe is polio-free.

It was formerly among the most dreaded illnesses in the US, but the threat was eliminated in the 1950s with the development of a vaccine. Even though polio is no longer present in the United States, visitors might still carry it with them.

Poliomyelitis is the abbreviation for it. It is a virus that quickly spreads among unvaccinated individuals. In its most extreme form, it can attack your brain and spinal cord, paralyzing you.

Anyone can contract polio, but children under the age of five are most at risk.

Chapter 2: Symptoms of polio

The majority of poliovirus carriers have no symptoms. Approximately 1 in 4 persons will experience symptoms that resemble the flu, such as:
unwell throat
- Being worn out
- uneasy stomach
- Fever
- Headache
- stiffness or back discomfort in the neck
- muscle tremor
- abdominal pain
- These "Nonparalytic Polio" symptoms, such as vomiting, frequently do not result in paralysis. Within ten days, they often disappear on their own.

A lesser percentage of persons experience "paralytic polio," a more severe form of

polio. If you have it, you will first have symptoms similar to the previous mild ones. In a week, you'll also begin to experience:
- A slowdown in reflexes
- Muscular weakness or excruciating pain
- Shaky limbs
- your legs experience a pins-and-needles sensation
- Arms, legs, or both paralyzed
- Meningitis (an infection in your brain, spinal cord, or both)
- If the breathing muscles you use become so weak that they stop functioning, polio can be fatal.

You could begin to experience various symptoms years after you recover from polio. You could have "post-polio syndrome," which includes:
- Breathing and swallowing issues
- muscle wasting
- Disturbances of sleep, such as sleep apnea

- Difficulty coping with low temperatures
- Acute flaccid myelitis (AFM), an uncommon but deadly disorder that likewise affects the neurological system and results in muscular weakness, is not the same as polio. AFM is sometimes referred to as having "polio-like" symptoms, however the virus is different.

Causes And Risk Factors For Polio

Any age can be affected by polio, although children under the age of five are most commonly affected.

A virus causes polio to spread. To contract the virus, you must have direct touch with it. Person-to-person interaction or coming into contact with a contaminated object might cause this. The virus resides in your intestines and throat while you have it.

Poliomyelitis Afterward

A whopping 40% of paralytic polio survivors may experience new symptoms 15 to 40 years after the initial infection. The post-polio syndrome symptoms include new, growing muscular weakening, extreme exhaustion, and pain in the muscles and joints.

Polio may lead to
Acute flaccid paralysis (AFP)
200 infections every year result in permanent paralysis, which generally affects the legs. The virus infecting the central nervous system and entering the bloodstream is what causes this. The virus kills the nerve cells that control muscular contraction as it replicates. Acute flaccid paralysis is a disorder in which the afflicted muscles become non-functional and the affected limb becomes floppy and lifeless (AFP).

Within 48 hours of the beginning, all instances of acute flaccid paralysis (AFP) in children under the age of fifteen are reported and tested for poliovirus.

Bulbar Polio

Quadriplegia is a more severe kind of paralysis that affects the abdominal, thorax, and trunk muscles. The poliovirus destroys the nerve cells in the brain stem in the most severe instances (bulbar polio), which impairs breathing and makes swallowing and speaking difficult. When their respiratory muscles are paralyzed, 5% to 10% of persons who are paralyzed pass away.

Bulbar polio patients in the 1940s and 1950s were kept alive and immobilized within "iron lungs" made of enormous metal cylinders that functioned like a pair of bellows to control their breathing. The positive pressure ventilator has largely taken the role of the iron lung in modern medicine, but it is still utilized.

Transmission

Person-to-person contact is how polio is transferred. The wild poliovirus that infects children enters the body through the mouth and grows in the gut. Then, through the feces, it is released into the environment, where it can quickly spread across a population, particularly under conditions of poor hygiene and sanitation. If enough kids receive the entire polio vaccine, the virus becomes extinct since it cannot infect any more vulnerable kids.

No matter their surroundings, young children who have not yet learned to use the bathroom are an easy source of transmission. When feces are present in food or beverages, polio can spread. Additionally, there is proof that flies can unintentionally spread the poliovirus from feces to meals.

Additionally, your kid risks contracting an infection if they put toys or other items in their mouth that have stools or other bodily fluids on them.

An infected individual can pass the virus on to others before symptoms appear and often 1 to 2 weeks afterward. The virus may remain active for several weeks in the intestines of an infected individual. When they contact food and drink with unclean hands, they run the risk of contaminating it.

taking in droplets from a polio patient's cough or sneeze. It's less typical to contract polio this way.

If you have polio in your body, you can still transmit it to others even if you don't show any symptoms.

The majority of poliovirus victims show no symptoms and are completely unaware of their infection. Before the first incidence of polio paralysis appears, these asymptomatic individuals can "silently" infect thousands of other individuals by carrying the virus in their intestines.

Because of this, the WHO views even one verified case of polio paralysis as evidence of an epidemic, particularly in nations where there aren't many instances.

Despite the fact that polio mostly affects children under the age of 5, anybody who has not had the polio vaccination is at significant risk.

Anyone who has not received the whole polio vaccination series is at danger since polio knows no boundaries. It is challenging to diagnose polio and stop the spread of the virus because for every instance of paralysis, there might be 200 (for poliovirus type 1) or 2,000 (for poliovirus type 2) children who are afflicted yet have no symptoms. People who are unvaccinated and reside in locations with low immunity levels are particularly at risk. Getting vaccinated is the greatest method to defend yourself and your family from polio. To keep everyone in the United States safe from polio, regular childhood immunization programs must maintain high vaccine coverage.

Allergies and polio risk factors
Nobody is aware of the reason why only a tiny fraction of infections result in paralysis. There are a number of significant risk factors that have been found to raise the possibility of paralysis in polio patients. These consist of:

- Immune dysfunction
- Tonsil removal during pregnancy (tonsillectomy)
- Intramuscular injections of drugs, etc.
- Injury from hard exercise

Chapter 3: Prevention and Treatment

I regret to inform you that there is no effective treatment for polio. The most effective method of polio prevention is vaccination. There are two vaccines that have been used successfully and safely in the United States since 2000: the inactivated polio vaccine (IPV) and the oral polio vaccine (OPV).

Volunteers may administer the oral form of the OPV vaccine. OPV prevents poliovirus transmission by promoting gut immunity, which benefits both the individual and the community.

An experienced healthcare professional must administer IPV via injection. Because IPV does not induce gut immunity and because immunized people can shed the virus in their stool if infected, it is unable to stop the spread of the virus in a community. IPV is incredibly effective at protecting individuals from serious disease brought on by poliovirus.

If you have polio, your doctor will prioritize your comfort and work to avoid developing any other health problems. Several remedies and resources for support include:

- Drugs that reduce pain (like ibuprofen)
- An oxygenator (a device that helps you breathe)
- Maintaining the function of your muscles with physical therapy
- For flu-like symptoms, bed rest and fluids
- antispasmodic drugs to ease muscle tension
- Urinary tract infection antibiotics
- A heating pad for aching and cramping muscles
- Adaptive braces

- Rehabilitation for the lungs to aid with lung issues
- Using a cane, wheelchair, or electric scooter as a mobility assistance

Polio Eradication

Although there is no treatment for polio, a vaccination gives your body the means to fend off the infection.

Thousands of individuals every year were paralyzed by the virus until the vaccine was developed in the 1950s. Fewer than 10 cases of polio were reported in the United States by the 1970s due to widespread vaccination.

The IPV vaccination is now given to children in the US in four doses, one at each of the following ages:

- 24 weeks
- One year
- Six to eighteen months

- Age group of 4 to 6 years

1. If you had the polio vaccination as a child and are now an adult, you should still be immune. The only times you might get a booster shot are if you intend to visit a nation where polio is still prevalent or if you interact often with polio sufferers.

2.

3. Your doctor can administer them if you missed any shots or are unsure. You'll have two doses spaced between 4 and 8 weeks, followed by a third shot between 6 and 12 months afterwards.

4. While the majority of the world is likewise free of polio, outbreaks of the virus have not been completely contained in Afghanistan, Nigeria, and Pakistan.

To eradicate polio, we must:

1. Identify and stop any new outbreaks as soon as possible.

2. Get whole cultures involved in the mission to reach every kid

3. Make specific arrangements to reach children in rural areas, conflict zones, and mobile and migratory communities.

4. The greatest national defense against polio is to strengthen regular vaccination.

5. Make sure sensitive surveillance is in place, especially in remote areas.

6. encourage governments to provide further public services to the most vulnerable citizens

7. Must continue to have the maximum degree of political support from national administrations and international organizations.

8. Make sure the necessary funding is available to complete the project.

It is advised that everyone obtain the entire course of polio vaccinations in order to be completely protected against the disease, even if they had contracted it as a child. Polioviruses come in three different types: type 1, type 2, and type 3. You are not immune to contracting the other varieties of polio if you have one type.

Since 2000, the sole polio vaccination administered in the US has been the inactivated polio vaccine (IPV), which offers protection from all three poliovirus strains.

Speak with your healthcare practitioner about being vaccinated if you haven't obtained all of the necessary doses or the polio vaccine.

If you or anybody in your family has gotten polio vaccination outside of the United States, be sure it complies with U.S. regulations and that you have proof that it shields you from all three kinds of polio, namely types 1, 2, and 3.

To be deemed completely vaccinated against polio, the documentation must state that you have had the age-appropriate polio vaccination series with either an inactivated polio vaccine, or IPV, or a trivalent oral polio vaccine, commonly known as tOPV. Two vaccinations that protect against all three polio forms include IPV and tOPV. The only polio vaccine used in the United States is IPV, which must be given in a series of three or four doses, depending on the age of the person who has to be immunized, if you have only gotten a bivalent OPV or bOPV, which only includes two types of polioviruses.

Only written documents with dates are accepted as proof of prior immunization. According to the U.S. schedule, everyone who lacks or just has dubious proof of their poliovirus immunization should get it again.

Talk with your healthcare practitioner as their recommendations for poliovirus immunization for you will depend on how many polio vaccines you have already gotten, which forms of polio vaccine you have had, and the time available until protection is needed.

Adults who completed the polio vaccination series as children and are going to travel to areas or countries with elevated risk of polio or have a higher risk for exposure to polio can receive a lifetime booster dose of IPV.

Talk with your healthcare practitioner about obtaining one lifetime booster of IPV.

Anyone who is not completely vaccinated against polio is at risk getting polio.
However, there are specific scenarios that place persons at elevated risk for exposure to polio such as:

Travelers who have recently visited polio endemic nations (Afghanistan and Pakistan) or countries suffering polio epidemics.
Laboratory and healthcare professionals who handle specimens that potentially contain polioviruses.

Healthcare personnel who are treating patients who potentially have polio or have direct contact with a person who could be infected with poliovirus.

People who are in contact with or care for a person who might be infected with polio or has been exposed to polio.

Unvaccinated adults whose children may be getting oral poliovirus vaccination while residing abroad

Talk with your healthcare practitioner to find out whether you may need a booster injection. Their advice for poliovirus immunization will depend on how many doses of polio vaccine you have already had and the time available until protection is needed

Allergies

The vaccine may cause an allergic reaction in some people. Typically, you'll notice any allergy symptoms between a few minutes and a few hours after developing them. In order to determine if you are allergic to the polio vaccine, look out for:

- Difficulty in breathing
- Weakness
- A raspy voice or wheezing
- A quick heartbeat
- Hives
- Dizziness
- If any of these symptoms apply to you, contact your doctor right away.

Allergies and polio risk factors

Nobody is aware of the reason why just a tiny fraction of infections result in paralysis. There are a number of significant risk factors that have been shown to raise the possibility of paralysis in polio patients. These consist of:

- Immunological dysfunction
- Tonsil removal during pregnancy (tonsillectomy)
- Intramuscular injections of drugs, etc.
- Injury from hard workout

Immunization Allergies

The immunization may cause an adverse response in some persons. Typically, you'll notice any allergy symptoms within a few minutes and a few hours after developing them. In order to determine if you are allergic to the polio vaccination, look out for:

- Difficulty in breathing

- Weakness
- A raspy voice or wheezing
- A quick heartbeat
- Hives
- Dizziness
- If any of these symptoms apply to you, contact your doctor right away.

What Measures Have You Taken Against Polio Today.